Natural Beauty Secrets

Easy Homemade Coconut & Essential Oil Recipes for Radiant Skin and Hair

Tara Evans

Just to say "thank you" for buying this book, I'd like to give you a bonus gift *absolutely free*

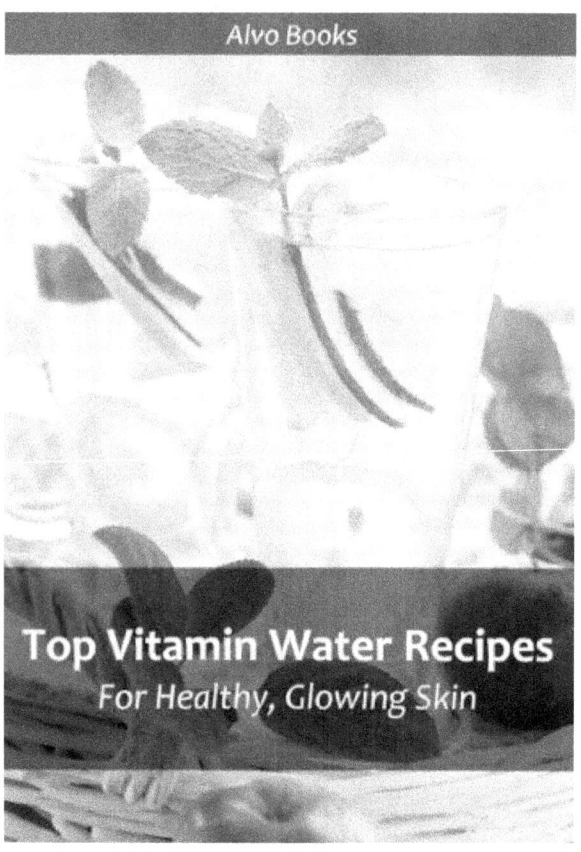

To claim your copy, go to:
www.alvobooks.com/naturalbeauty

First Published in 2014 by Alvo Books

Copyright © Tara Evans

This book is presented solely for educational and entertainment purposes. For diagnosis or treatment of any medical problem, consult your own physician. The publisher and author are not responsible for any specific health or allergy needs that may require medical supervision and are not liable for any damages or negative consequences from any treatment, action, application or preparation, to any person reading or following the information in this book. Although the author and publisher have made every effort to ensure that the information in this book was correct at press time, the author and publisher do not assume and hereby disclaim any liability to any party for any loss, damage, or disruption caused by errors or omissions, whether such errors or omissions result from negligence, accident, or any other cause.

Contents

Introduction

Some of you may be wondering what all the hype is about essential oils. They have come into the light more frequently in recent years as people are becoming more aware about the harsh chemicals in the skin products they use. This book provides coconut and essential oil recipes for simple, homemade skin care products to help you eliminate those harsh chemicals and pamper yourself at the same time! The natural ingredients are all easy to find and I've made sure the recipes only use a few basic ingredients to keep them as economical as possible.

Now, to answer some of your questions:

What are essential oils?

Essential oils are produced directly from plants. They have many medicinal properties, and contain antifungal, antibacterial and antiviral components. Try to think of these ingredients as the 'essence' of the plants they come from. They are highly potent and a little definitely goes a long way! Before purchasing any products, make sure you are actually buying essential oil. Any product that is listed as a perfume, blend or fragrance will most likely have a synthetic base (which is what we are trying to avoid!).

How can I safely use essential oils?

Most essential oils are too potent to be used directly on the skin. They are generally paired with a carrier oil. A carrier oil dilutes the potency of the essential oil and makes it safe to use directly on skin. Some examples of carrier oils are grape seed oil, sweet almond oil, avocado oil, jojoba oil and olive oil. Carrier oils are generally packed with their own nutrients to help nourish the skin.

Are there any warnings for essential oils?

1. It is not recommended to use essential oils on babies or small children. Their skin is generally much thinner and more sensitive.

2. Keep in mind that if you have any food allergies, you will also be allergic to the essential oil counterpart.

3. If your chosen carrier oil is almond oil, or any other 'nut' oil, beware of coming into contact with people with nut allergies. In extreme cases of nut allergy, there is the possibility of causing a reaction from the residual oil left on the skin.

4. Avoid using essential oils if you are pregnant or nursing.

5. Always test a small area of the skin before using your new product.

6. Avoid contact with eyes.

Why is coconut oil good for my skin?

Not only is coconut oil a natural substance, but it is packed full of vitamins and antioxidants that are super beneficial for the skin, and doesn't contain any harsh chemicals or synthetic ingredients.

Coconut oil is not only naturally moisturizing for your hair, skin and nails, but it also has antifungal and antibacterial properties as well! It's incredibly versatile and can be used to make amazing lip balms, hair treatments, soaps, scrubs, creams and even deodorant. Coconut oil truly is nature's best beauty secret.

Where can I get the ingredients for these recipes?

Most of these recipes are available at your local supermarket, or health food/supplement store. If you don't have easy access to a wide variety of items, ordering online is also a great option. However, make sure you are purchasing organic ingredients from a reputable company. There are a lot of products available online that are made from someone's home, without proper documentation of the methods or ingredients used. Here is a list of the main ingredients included in this book:

1. Coconut oil – Unrefined and organic coconut oil is preferred because it retains much of the original plant's vitamins and nutrients.

2. Coconut milk – Any coconut milk will do fine, as long as it's pure!

3. Glycerin soap base – Located at most craft stores in the soap making section, or you can purchase online.

4. Essential oils – Most essential oils should be packaged in dark glass bottles. They need to be stored out of direct sunlight and intense heat. If you live nearby a health food/supplement store, you may prefer to shop for your essential oils there. This would be the preferred option, that way you can discuss the different brands with the salesperson and find which essential oil company works best for you. The other option is ordering your essential oils online. As good quality essential oils are a bit of an investment, I've made sure that this book keeps the number of oils you need to buy to a minimum, and I've also used the most readily available oils.

5. Grape seed oil – Grape seed oil is not as moisturizing as olive oil, but is wonderful on the skin and tends to absorb a little better. It's also lighter. If you can't find grape seed oil at the supermarket, your best bet is to ask at a health food/supplement store or buy it online. Just make sure you're buying 100% pure, or unrefined, grape seed oil, which means there are no additives or chemicals.

6. Olive oil – Highly moisturizing! You can find olive oil at your local supermarket in the cooking section.

7. Witch hazel – This is an astringent made from the witch hazel plant. It has good anti-inflammatory, anti-bacterial and anti-fungal properties. You can usually find witch hazel astringent at the supermarket, or health food/supplement shop.

8. Aloe vera – You can find the bottled gel at the supermarket in the skincare section, or if you have an aloe vera plant in your house (which is great for purifying the air of your home!) you can take cuttings from the plant.

9. Vitamin E – For these recipes you can either buy Vitamin E liquid, or the gel capsules (sold in the vitamin section at the grocery store). If you go for the capsule option, you will have to pierce the shell with a needle and squeeze out the liquid.

Now that we've covered some of the basics, let's get started with some quick and easy recipes!

Glycerin Soap Bars

Glycerin soap bars are easy and fun to make. You can find 'melt and pour' kits at your local craft store that will have the glycerin soap base and molds, or you can buy different varieties of glycerin bases (aloe, shea butter, goat's milk, oatmeal and plain glycerin bases are the most common) and use old muffin tins for your soap molds. I find it easier to have an extra muffin tin to use just for skincare and craft purposes to avoid any cross contamination with your cookware. Once soaps are fully hardened, pop them out of the molds and enjoy for yourself, or you can package creatively for beautiful gifts!

Luscious Vanilla, Coconut and Coffee Soap

Coffee grounds and ground cinnamon both have antioxidants and act to exfoliate your skin. Coconut milk is naturally moisturizing and is packed full of vitamins. You can find coconut milk and coconut oil at most food stores, just aim to buy organic!

Ingredients:
1. 8 ounces plain glycerin soap base
2. ¼ cup coconut milk
3. ¼ cup coffee grounds (used grounds work well)
4. ½ cup coconut oil
5. 1 teaspoon pure vanilla extract

Directions:
1. Melt the glycerin in either a double boiler on the stove or in a microwave-safe container using one minute increments. I don't have a double boiler, so I make my own with an old pot filled with a few inches of water and melt the glycerin in a pint sized Mason jar. (Just make sure you have pot holders available, as the Mason jar will get hot!)

2. Add in the coconut oil and coconut milk. Mix well. Coconut oil is solid at 76 degrees Fahrenheit, so if you decided to use the microwave, you may need to put the mixture back in to heat up a little more.

3. Stir in the coffee grounds and vanilla extract until evenly dispersed.

4. Pour into molds and let set for 30 minutes. Once fully hardened, pop the soap out of the molds and enjoy, or package creatively for gifts!

Lemon Zest and Shea Butter Soap

Ingredients:

1. 8 ounces shea butter glycerin soap base
2. ½ cup coconut oil
3. 2 teaspoons lemon zest (for color and scent)
4. 20 drops lemon essential oil

Directions:

1. Melt the glycerin in either a double boiler on the stove or in a microwave-safe container using one minute increments. I don't have a double boiler, so I make my own with an old pot filled with a few inches of water and melt the glycerin in a pint sized Mason jar. (Just make sure you have pot holders available, as the Mason jar will get hot!)

2. Add in the coconut oil (coconut oil is solid at 76 degrees Fahrenheit, so if you decided to use the microwave, you may need to put the mixture back in to heat up a little more). Mix together.

3. Mix in the lemon zest and essential oil.

4. Pour into molds and let set for 30 minutes.

Soothing Aloe and Eucalyptus Soap

Aloe and eucalyptus are both great for relieving sun burns and skin inflammation.

Ingredients:
1. 8 ounces aloe glycerin soap base
2. ¼ cup coconut oil
3. 1 or 2 cuttings from aloe plant (or 1 teaspoon aloe gel)
4. 20 drops eucalyptus essential oil

Directions:
1. Melt the glycerin in either a double boiler on the stove or in a microwave-safe container using one minute increments. I don't have a double boiler, so I make my own with an old pot filled with a few inches of water and melt the glycerin in a pint sized Mason jar. (Just make sure you have pot holders available, as the Mason jar will get hot!)

2. Add in the coconut oil (coconut oil is solid at 76 degrees Fahrenheit, so if you decided to use the microwave, you may need to put the mixture back in to heat up a little more). Mix together.

3. Squeeze out the gel from the aloe cuttings and add in, along with the eucalyptus essential oil.

4. Pour into molds and let set for 30 minutes.

Exfoliating Coconut Oil, Oatmeal and Goat's Milk Soap

For this recipe, the oatmeal acts to mildly exfoliate your skin and the cinnamon has great antioxidants!

Ingredients:
1. 8 ounces goat's milk glycerin soap base
2. ¼ cup oatmeal, blended lightly
3. ¼ cup coconut oil
4. 2 teaspoons ground cinnamon

Directions:
1. Melt the glycerin in either a double boiler on the stove or in a microwave-safe container using one minute increments. I don't have a double boiler, so I make my own with an old pot filled with a few inches of water and melt the glycerin in a pint sized Mason jar. (Just make sure you have pot holders available, as the Mason jar will get hot!)

2. Add in the coconut oil (coconut oil is solid at 76 degrees Fahrenheit, so if you decided to use the microwave, you may need to put the mixture back in to heat up a little more).

3. Add in the lightly blended oatmeal and ground cinnamon and mix thoroughly.

4. Pour into molds and let set for 30 minutes.

Peppermint Milk Soap

Peppermint essential oil helps relieve stress and sore muscles leaving you feeling refreshed! Paired with exfoliating sugar and moisturizing goat's milk, this recipe is great after a long day.

Ingredients:
1. 8 ounces Goat's Milk glycerin soap base
2. ½ cup granulated sugar
3. 25 drops peppermint essential oil

Directions:
1. Melt the glycerin in either a double boiler on the stove or in a microwave-safe container using one minute increments. I don't have a double boiler, so I make my own with an old pot filled with a few inches of water and melt the glycerin in a pint sized Mason jar. (Just make sure you have pot holders available, as the Mason jar will get hot!)

2. Add in the sugar and peppermint essential oil.

3. Pour into molds and let set for 30 minutes.

Hair Products

Coconut oil is a great way to moisturize your hair and provides a beautiful natural shine. It's also great for controlling frizzy hair. For each recipe you will want a reusable container that is safe to store in the shower. (Preferably plastic, glass gets slippery in the shower and could accidentally break!) Coconut oil is generally solid at room temperature, but does melt at around 76 degrees Fahrenheit (about 24 degrees Celsius). If you notice your mixture has a hardened layer, hold the container under warm water for a few minutes and it will melt quickly.

Coconut Milk Shampoo with Lavender and Rosemary

This recipe calls for liquid castile soap. Real, authentic castile soap is made from vegetable or olive oils. It is free of synthetic materials and harsh chemicals. Make sure when purchasing that it is made from natural ingredients and doesn't have any extra additives. Lavender and rosemary essential oils will help you relax and reduce stress. They both have antibacterial properties as well!

Ingredients:
1. ½ cup coconut milk (any brand works, as long as it's pure)
2. ¾ cup liquid castile soap
3. 1 teaspoon grape seed oil
4. 15 drops lavender essential oil
5. 15 drops rosemary essential oil

Directions:
1. Mix together all the ingredients in your reusable container.

2. Massage into your hair like normal (this shampoo may not foam as much as your normal shampoo, since it doesn't have the added synthetic foaming ingredients).

3. Then condition your hair as normal. (The ingredients will separate, so make sure you shake well before each use.)

Coconut Oil Conditioner with Lavender and Rosemary

This recipe is great for all hair types, but especially for dry hair. If you have more regular/oily hair you may only want to apply to the lower half of your hair or the ends.

Note: coconut oil will most likely solidify between uses, so make sure to let the container heat up under warm water before each use. Lavender and rosemary essential oils will help you relax and reduce stress. They both have antibacterial properties as well!

Ingredients:
1. 1 cup melted coconut oil
2. 1 tablespoon grape seed oil
3. 1 tablespoon olive oil
4. 15 drops lavender essential oil
5. 15 drops rosemary essential oil

Directions:
1. Melt the coconut oil in a microwave-safe container using 30 second increments.

2. Pour the coconut oil and other ingredients into your chosen reusable container and mix well.

3. Apply the conditioner like normal, allowing it to sit on your hair for a few minutes before thoroughly rinsing

out. (The ingredients will separate, so make sure you shake well before each use.)

Honey, Apple Cider Vinegar and Coconut Oil Hair Mask

Honey and coconut oil will help smooth your hair and hold in moisture. The apple cider vinegar will remove build up on the hair from commercial and synthetic products. This mask will leave your hair with a beautiful shine! Use once a week or as needed.

Note: Honey may lighten your hair over extended periods of time, so I wouldn't recommend using this mask more than once or twice a week.

Ingredients:
1. 1 cup melted coconut oil
2. ½ cup apple cider vinegar
3. 1 cup honey

Directions:
1. Melt the coconut oil in a microwave-safe container using 30 second increments.

2. Pour the melted coconut oil into your reusable container.

3. Add in the apple cider vinegar and honey, mixing well.

4. Massage the mask onto your hair and scalp and let it sit for 30 minutes. Then shampoo and condition like normal.

(Make sure to shake the bottle well before each use, as the ingredients will separate.)

Replenishing Coconut and Olive Oil Hair Mask

This hair mask is perfect for dry hair and scalps!

Note: Honey may lighten your hair over extended periods of time, so I wouldn't recommend using this mask more than once or twice a week.

Ingredients:
1. 1 cup melted coconut oil
2. ½ cup olive oil
3. ¼ cup honey

Directions:
1. Melt the coconut oil in microwave-safe container using 30 second increments.

2. Pour the melted coconut oil into your reusable container.

3. Mix in the olive oil and honey.

4. Apply generously to your hair and scalp. Let the mixture sit for 20-30 minutes before showering like normal. (The ingredients will separate, so make sure you shake well before using.)

Liquid Castile Body Washes

These recipes call for liquid castile soap. Castile soap is made from olive or vegetable oils, and shouldn't contain any extra chemical additives. It is gentle on the skin, and tends to lather a little more than glycerin soap. You will most likely find it at your local supermarket, but if not, it's pretty inexpensive to order it online too!

Everyday Coconut Milk Body Wash

This recipe is super simple, and doesn't have any added scent. It's great for sensitive skin or people who dislike perfumes.

Ingredients:
1. ½ cup coconut milk
2. 1 cup castile soap
3. ¼ cup grape seed oil

Directions:
1. Mix all the ingredients together in your reusable plastic container.

2. Shake well before each use, as the ingredients will separate.

Moisturizing Honey Body Wash

This is one of my favorite body washes because it's both luscious and refreshing.

Ingredients:
1. ½ cup coconut milk
2. ¼ cup grape seed oil
3. 2 tablespoons honey
4. 1 cup castile soap
5. 25 drops grapefruit essential oil

Directions:
1. Mix together the coconut milk, grape seed oil and castile soap in your reusable container.

2. Add in the honey and essential oils.

3. Shake well before each use, as the ingredients will separate.

Soothing Body Wash

This is a great choice after a long stressful day as the lavender and peppermint oils will soothe and relax.

Ingredients:
1. ½ cup coconut milk
2. 3 tablespoons olive oil
3. 1 cup castile soap
4. 15 drops peppermint essential oil
5. 20 drops lavender essential oil

Directions:
1. Mix together the coconut milk, olive oil and castile soap in your reusable container.

2. Add in the peppermint and lavender essential oils.

3. Shake well before each use.

Invigorating Peppermint Wash

For a minty pick me up, try this peppermint wash!

Ingredients:
1. 3 tablespoons olive oil
2. 2 tablespoons grape seed oil
3. 1 cup castile soap
4. 25 drops peppermint essential oil

Directions:
1. Mix together the olive oil, grape seed oil and castile soap to your reusable container.

2. Add in the peppermint oil.

3. Shake well before each use.

Natural Lip Products

Nourish your lips with these natural and moisturizing lip balms! Each recipe makes enough for a few containers, so make sure you have several clean, reusable containers on hand. You can use cleaned make up containers, empty roll up stick containers, or even left over mint tins. You'll have your friends and family fighting over who gets the extra lip balm!

Note: Beeswax is very difficult to clean off, so make sure you use a preparation container that you don't mind having a slight residue on. I use old pots or glass bowls that I don't use for cooking anymore for all of my homemade skin care recipes.

Tinted Moisturizing Lip Stain

Ingredients:
1. 1 cup coconut oil
2. ½ cup beeswax
3. 1-2 cuttings of aloe vera leaves (or 1 teaspoon aloe vera gel)
4. ¼ teaspoon pure cocoa powder
5. Pinch of ground cinnamon (or drop or two of red natural food coloring)

Directions:
1. In a microwave-safe container, melt the beeswax using 1 minute increments. (You can also use a double boiler on your stove top, like we did to make the soaps.)

2. Add in the coconut oil and honey. You may need to heat the mixture for another minute to make sure everything is in liquid form and mixed thoroughly.

3. Squeeze in the gel from aloe vera leaves

4. Mix in the cocoa powder and cinnamon. You can add more depending on how dark or red you want your lip stain to be. Remember that a little goes a long way, so add in just a little at a time.

5. The mixture will be hot, so let it cool for a minute or so before carefully pouring into containers.

6. Allow the lip stain to cool for 30 minutes.

Sweet Orange Lip Balm

Ingredients:
1. 1 cup coconut oil
2. 2 tablespoons honey
3. ½ cup beeswax
4. 5 drops vitamin E
5. 20 drops sweet orange essential oil

Directions:
1. In a microwave-safe container, melt the beeswax using 1 minute increments.

2. Add in the coconut oil and honey. You may need to heat the mixture for another minute to make sure everything is in liquid form and mixed thoroughly.

3. Finally, add in the sweet orange essential oil and vitamin E.

4. The mixture will be hot, so let it cool for a minute or so before carefully pouring into containers.

5. Let the lip balm cool for 30 minutes.

Basic Coconut Oil Lip Balm

Ingredients:

1. 1 cup coconut oil
2. ½ cup beeswax
3. 5 drops vitamin E

Directions:

1. In a microwave-safe container, melt the beeswax using 1 minute increments.

2. Add in the coconut oil. You may need to heat the mixture for another minute to make sure everything is in liquid form and mixed thoroughly.

3. Finally, mix in the vitamin E. The mixture will be hot, so let it cool for a minute or so before carefully pouring into containers.

4. Allow the lip balm to set for 30 minutes.

Natural Peppermint Beeswax Lip Balm

Ingredients:

1. 1 cup coconut oil
2. ½ cup beeswax
3. 2 tablespoons honey
4. 15 drops peppermint essential oil

Directions:

1. In a microwave-safe container, melt the beeswax using 1 minute increments.

2. Add in the coconut oil and honey. You may need to heat the mixture for another minute to make sure everything is in liquid form and mixed thoroughly.

3. Finally, add in the peppermint essential oil. The mixture will be hot, so let it cool for a minute or so before carefully pouring into containers.

4. Allow the lip balm to cool for 30 minutes.

Moisturizing Lip Scrub

This is a great scrub to use during the winter months, when your lips dry out and get chapped.

Ingredients:
1. 1 teaspoon coconut oil
2. 1 teaspoon brown/white sugar
3. 1 teaspoon honey

Directions:
1. In a microwave-safe container, melt the coconut oil using 30 second increments.

2. Add in the honey. Mix in the brown or white sugar.

3. Gently rub the lip scrub onto your lips and let it sit for 5 minutes, then wipe off with a warm wash cloth.

4. This recipe makes enough scrub for several uses, so store in an airtight container between uses.

Body Scrubs

Naturally exfoliate and soften your skin with these recipes! They can be kept in reusable plastic containers, or add a ribbon to a mason jar and give away for gifts.

Zesty Coconut Oil and Epsom Salt Scrub

Ingredients:

1. 1 cup Epsom salt
2. 1 cup coconut oil
3. 1 cup grape seed oil
4. 20 drops lemon essential oil
5. 2 teaspoons lemon zest (for coloring and added scent)

Directions:

1. Melt the coconut oil in a microwave-safe container.

2. Add in the Epsom salt and lemon zest, followed by the lemon essential oil.

3. Allow the scrub to warm up under the shower to melt the coconut oil before each use, and gently massage into your skin while showering.

Coconut Oil, Coffee and Brown Sugar Exfoliating Bar

While everyone loves this exfoliating bar, it's also great for men because it doesn't have any 'girly' scents. It's a great way to trick guys into exfoliating without them even realizing it!

Ingredients:
1. 1 cup brown sugar
2. ½ cup coconut oil
3. ½ cup beeswax
4. ½ cup coffee grounds
5. 20 drops nutmeg essential oil
6. 20 drops pure vanilla extract

Directions:
1. In a microwave-safe container, melt the beeswax using one minute increments.

2. Add in the coconut oil, coffee grounds and brown sugar, making sure everything is evenly incorporated.

3. Mix in the nutmeg essential oil and pure vanilla extract.

4. Let the mixture harden in a muffin tin or soap molds for 30 minutes.

5. Store the bars in an airtight container to hold in the scent.

Spicy Citrus Sugar Scrub

Ingredients:
1. 1 cup white/brown sugar
2. 1 cup coconut oil
3. ½ cup grape seed oil
4. 2 teaspoons orange zest
5. 20 drops sweet orange essential oil
6. 15 drops clove essential oil

Directions:
1. Melt the coconut oil in a microwave-safe container using one minute increments.

2. Mix in the grape seed oil, white or brown sugar, and orange zest.

3. Add in the essential oils.

4. Allow the scrub to warm up under the shower to melt the coconut oil before each use, and gently massage into your skin while showering.

If you want an even more citrusy scent, add in a few drops of grapefruit essential oil.

Extras

There are just so many amazing things you can make with coconut and essential oils, so I've included some special bonus recipes for you!

Refreshing and Moisturizing Body Spray

I love using this refreshing spray in summer – not only does it smell great, it's also nice and refreshing.

Ingredients:
1. ¼ cup filtered water
2. 2 teaspoons vegetable glycerin (liquid)
3. 1 ½ teaspoons grape seed oil
4. 20 drops peppermint essential oil
5. 3 ounce pump spray bottle

Directions:
1. Mix together the filtered water, glycerin and grape seed oil.

2. Add in the essential oils.

3. Pour into a pump spray bottle.

4. Make sure to shake well before you each use. Best if used right after showering!

Nourishing Coconut Oil Lotion Bar

Use this bar at the end of your shower or bath to moisturize.

Ingredients:
1. 1 cup coconut oil
2. 1 cup beeswax
3. ½ cup shea butter
4. ¼ cup grape seed oil
5. 25 drops clove essential oil

Directions:
1. Melt the beeswax in microwave-safe container using one minute increments.

2. Add in the coconut oil, shea butter and grape seed oil.

3. Mix in the clove essential oil.

4. Pour into muffin tins or soap molds and let it harden for 30 minutes.

Natural Deodorant

Store bought antiperspirants are packed full of harmful chemicals, and most natural deodorants are expensive and don't always work well. This recipe is all natural and isn't expensive to make! Keep in mind that this is a deodorant, not an antiperspirant, so you will still sweat. Sweating is how the body naturally gets rid of toxins from the body, and is important for healthy functioning. This natural deodorant will keep you smelling fresh.

Ingredients:
1. 2 tablespoons coconut oil
2. 1 tablespoon beeswax
3. 2 tablespoons baking soda
4. 2 ½ tablespoons cornstarch
5. 10 drops lavender essential oil
6. 20 drops bergamot essential oil

Directions:
1. Melt the beeswax and coconut oil in a microwave-safe container.

2. Slowly mix in the baking soda and cornstarch.

3. Incorporate the essential oils.

4. Scoop your deodorant into your chosen container. You can reuse your old deodorant roll up sticks; however, if

you live in a warmer climate, it's best to use a plastic or glass container and rub the deodorant under your arms since the coconut oil will melt at 76 degrees Fahrenheit (24 degrees Celsius) and above.

Natural Hand Sanitizer

This hand sanitizer recipe is packed with antibacterial, antifungal and antioxidant properties! It also smells wonderful!

Ingredients:
1. 3 tablespoons aloe vera gel
2. ½ teaspoon grape seed oil
3. 1 tablespoon witch hazel
4. 20 drops tea tree essential oil
5. 15 drops rosemary essential oil
6. 15 drops lavender essential oil
7. 15 drops clove essential oil
8. 4 ounce pump spray bottle

Directions:
1. Mix together all ingredients and pour into the pump spray bottle.

2. Make sure to shake well before each use.

Conclusion

If you're looking for new ways to cut out harsh chemicals from your daily life and want to live more organically, then making your own natural skin care and beauty products with essential oils and coconut oil is the way to go! Treat yourself every day with your new beauty secrets – and don't forget to share with your friends and family!

Can I Ask You a Favor?

I'm so glad you enjoyed this book enough to make it all the way to the end and I hope you've found it really useful. If you liked the book, would you be open to leaving an honest review? That would really help out other people who are looking for a book on the topic and it also helps us as a small, independent publisher.

To leave a review on the US site, go to www.amazon.com/dp/B00IGJ8ZOA, otherwise you can leave a review on the relevant Amazon page in your country.

Thank you!

www.ingramcontent.com/pod-product-compliance
Lightning Source LLC
Chambersburg PA
CBHW070230290526
45789CB00004B/1568